The Keto Collagen Diet

Discover the Benefits of Bone Broth and Collagen with Ketogenic Diet to Help You Lose Weight, Cure Keto Flu, Improve Gut Health, and Reverse Aging

Kendall Arrison

Table of Contents

Introduction

Let me start by saying that I appreciate you taking the time to select this book out of all the other options that you had. I can assure you that within this book, we will be doing a deep dive into a subject which is not covered often enough in other books where they try to overload you with information about all the different things you could try. I will be doing so from the viewpoint of personal experience and sharing with you the details of my journey wherever possible.

When I first heard about the ketogenic diet and the potential health benefits it could deliver, I have to say I was supremely skeptical. I was at the stage of my journey, perhaps much the same as you are now, where I felt like I had tried every diet, pill, meditation app, and cross-fit membership available, and for some reason, my overall health was still coming up short. I was lethargic, bloated, and low energy - and if that is how you are currently feeling, then let me start by saying that I understand completely! With the amount of information overload that we have through fitness programs, recommended diets, Instagram fitness influencers, and "fit-tubers", it is easy to fall into the trap of overwhelm and analysis paralysis. And even when I then did settle on one particular diet that seemed to work for me, there was still a mountain of information.

The extremes of the ketogenic diet are not for the faint-hearted, and it is not recommended as a first step on the weight loss journey. You should already have a regular workout regimen and a reasonably healthy eating routine under your belt before trying out keto and particularly the bone broth fast that we will go through in this book. If you are not at that stage yet, please try and incorporate some of the collagen and keto style benefits into your diet, gradually reducing carbs and increasing your collagen intake first before going full keto. I had been on the weight loss journey with varying success and had reached a plateau with my weight and my energy levels. I think it was only out of sheer necessity and desperation that I then turned to keto, and when I speak to other people who have found success with the keto lifestyle, that is a very similar story. When I did finally decide to give it a try, what I found was remarkable. Not only was it a holistic approach to weight loss, the extent of which I hadn't seen before, but it was also a diet that I found fascinating due to the scientific aspects of it. It opened my eyes to understanding my body in a way I had not done before. I became obsessed. I would regularly spend my time researching and reading up on all aspects of the keto lifestyle. While I found the information and support networks available to be of exceptionally high quality, I did find some areas to be slightly lacking in information. Particularly about the dreaded 'keto flu'. I struggled to find any practical advice on how to physically overcome this, deal with the symptoms, and understand the physical changes in my body during this time. I suffered tremendously through the keto flu, and that was mostly due to the lack of information that I had, which extended the flu period much longer than I needed to experience. I then discovered bone broth and the miracle properties that it contained. I started to look into how that could be used to help me overcome my issues with the keto flu. It is not just to minimize the symptoms of what I had experienced but also to provide a healthy and effective kickstart to people trying out the keto diet for the first time.

When I started to feel confident about the information I was researching, this then started my journey into developing and delivering the information to a wider audience. I want to share the benefits of what I had discovered. Which has led me right to this point of you reading this book right now, for which I am eternally grateful. I aim to hopefully contribute an integral part of the keto ecosystem by showing more people that this diet and lifestyle is not something to be feared. It can open doors to an amazing new life and health that you never knew existed.

I started looking into the impact it was proven to have on skin and even cellulite. Once I made it a regular part of my wellness routine, I also discovered for myself the immense benefits of using it to combat the keto flu. If you think that there is no need for a whole book just to focus on one adverse symptom of the ketogenic diet, then I can say for absolute certainty that you have never had the keto flu. Once you have experienced it and how devastating it can be to your plans, you will be chasing down encyclopedias to read if it would get rid of the symptoms. With the use of this book, you will never have to experience the side effects to the same level that I did because this book is full of tips, recipes, and strategies. Also, you will learn about that life-saving bone broth to make sure that your journey into keto is as happy, healthy, and effective as it can be.

I have also included my own 3-day collagen meal plan and bone broth fast to help you kick start your keto journey. These recipes can be used throughout the period that you decide to continue with the keto diet. If you are in the transition period, this will help immensely with symptoms of keto flu. There is never a wrong time to eat healthily and consume extra collagen, so even if you are just dipping your toe in the water and you are not ready to dive deeply into the ketogenic waters just yet, try incorporating some of the delicious recipes from my meal plans into your daily life. I am confident that you will start seeing noticeable results even from just taking that small step.

I am so honored to be part of your journey as you explore this fascinating lifestyle in more detail. I look forward to discussing the aspects of both collagen and bone broth in the next few chapters. My goal is to help you look into other areas of the ketogenic diet that might not be widely covered. I will try to help by sharing with you parts of my journey and by hopefully making you feel that you are not in this alone. All your hard work will be rewarded with the health, lifestyle, and body of your dreams. Thank you for choosing me as your guide for this process as I know there are plenty of competing titles out there, and if you are ready, then let us get started!

Chapter 1: Why Keto Collagen is like Keto on Steroids?

As with any book that takes a deep dive into a particular subject, I think it is crucial for us to, first of all, take a step back and look at the broader understanding, awareness, definition, and parameters of the ketogenic diet. We will then go into more detail about the benefits of collagen in particular and start to look at what bone broth is and exactly why it is so beneficial. But to understand the benefits, it is essential for us to, first of all, to establish exactly what the ketogenic diet is and why it can be so impactful and transformational when used properly.

In this chapter, I will also introduce you to the wonderful healing properties of bone broth. For the uninitiated, I completely understand why the term 'bone broth' might have you worried, but honestly, I cannot stress enough just how beneficial this is to your success with the ketogenic diet. With this book, I hope to at least encourage you to try it, and then I know that once you experience the benefits for yourself, you won't need any more persuading to keep it as a regular part of your diet.

The Fundamentals

The basic fundamental principles of the ketogenic diet align very closely with other low-carb, high-fat diets such as Atkins. But it goes a step further by applying what could be considered a more scientific approach. If you take something like the Atkins diet to the extreme and follow a diet that is so low in carbs that they are rendered entirely ineffective on your system, then your body goes into a state known as ketosis. This is a metabolic state where your body is almost starved of glucose so instead it burns fat for energy, resulting in residual acids being left in your system which are referred to as ketones. The reason for doing this is because your body runs much more efficiently when burning fat rather than having to work through the usually slower process of using carbohydrates for energy.

Digestion is the biggest drain on energy for the human body, and when all of your energy is coming from high-carb processed foods, or artificial sugar, which is converted through the pancreas, you are putting your body under the continuous pressure of boom and bust type energy cycles. Slow-release carbs that are found in products like fruit, squash, and sweet potato are the friendliest carbs for your system to handle. That is not surprising when you think about the difference between something that is eaten pretty much in its exact natural state and something that is concocted in a factory, doused with additives to make it last longer, stuffed into a packaging and stays on a shelf for months. Any food with a shelf life of over a year should be giving you absolute red flags as to what is in that food to make it last so long. Our bodies are supposed to eat foods in their natural state or as close to their natural state as possible, which is why diets like ketogenic and the paleo diet are so popular.

The downside is it becomes a challenging state for your body to stay in all the time. Most food and drink that we regularly consume in our modern lives would kick us immediately out of the ketogenic state. If you are used to a diet that is high in sugar, then the chances of you naturally staying in a ketogenic state are very low. Even with the recipes and foods prescribed as part of the keto diet, it can still be a problematic method to follow, and a lot of people find themselves only doing keto for short bursts of time, and implementing regular breaks where they can pick up some of their regular eating habits.

This is where it becomes vitally important to start looking at remedies, supplements, and support systems to ensure that staying in a ketogenic state becomes easier, as well as facilitating a smooth transition in and out of the ketogenic state when required. That is why, in this book, we will be looking particularly at how to alleviate the symptoms of keto flu to enable you the smooth transition of being able to access the ketogenic state as regularly as you wish. A lot of diet experts strongly advise that you only follow keto intermittently and that you return to more regular eating at more frequent intervals. Likewise, many keto enthusiasts stay in a keto state all the time. Personally, for me, I use it as a way to kick start other health and diet practices, and I usually don't stay in a ketogenic state for longer than a few weeks without taking a break. As with anything, it is good not to become too obsessed. And I enjoy a night out socializing and a cold glass of wine as much as anyone, so try and not let it overtake your life to the point where you are not enjoying the fantastic results that you are getting.

Collagen and the Keto Diet

Collagen is becoming very popular these days both in the health world and the beauty world, which is surprising as it has always been known to have been important for our health, skin, nails, and hair. We are now seeing it much more often in supplements, in beauty packs, and spa treatments. So, what exactly is collagen? And why is it so important for the ketogenic diet and in particular, what is the relation to bone broth, which sounds about as far away from a luxury Beverly Hills spa treatment as you could possibly get.

In later chapters, I will talk you through exactly why it is so beneficial and how to implement it properly within your keto regime. For now, I think it is important to understand first of all, precisely what collagen is.

Collagen is a structural protein found in the body. The word collagen is obtained from the greek word for 'glue' (kólla) and 'gen' which means to produce. This is because in ancient times, they used horse collagen to make glue. Collagen is the main ingredient of the body's connective tissue. It means that it is essentially what binds a lot of your body together. Connective tissue is one of the main types of tissue found in the human body (the others being epithelial tissue, muscle tissue, and nervous tissue). Collagen is found in bones, muscles, and skin. So by increasing and strengthening your levels of collagen, you can drastically improve joint health and achieve younger-looking skin. Younger looking skin and decreased cellulite were definitely the two health benefits that got me reading further. It is often very easy to overlook the parts of our body that we don't see, so another great positive for the keto diet is even just the awareness that it brings to how our bodies function and develop. I certainly found my research getting a lot more scientific than when I had looked at other diets that simply revolved around counting calories.

As we age, the collagen in the sub-layers of our skin stops binding so well with the elastin, and it can lead to loose skin, which causes cellulite and wrinkles. Elastin gives connective tissue some degree of elasticity. That is the reason why a baby's skin is able to return to its original position when it is poked or pinch, compare that to poking a wrinkled face. These are the most visible signs of collagen deficiency. Collagen also provides important protective layers for vital organs such as the kidneys. So if you are concerned about the reduction in collagen levels being visible on your thighs, just imagine what damage could be caused by not having sufficient collagen levels for your internal organs.

There are different types of collagen, although you will likely only ever come across a few of them when you are researching collagen for keto diet and regular use. In fact, there are 16 different types of collagen - with types I, II, and III being the ones most prevalent in our system. In general terms, we can think about Type I being related to our skin, eyes, nerve tissue, bone tissue, ligaments, artery walls, and knee joint. Type I is the most abundant type of collagen, making up 90% of all collagen in the body. Type II being most prominent in hyaline cartilage that can be found in the nose, ears, and larynx. Type III is found in skin and blood vessels. It is commonly used for gut healing and it helps improve the skin's elasticity together with Type I.

What is Bone Broth?

Bone broth is pretty much exactly as described. It is a soup-like mixture made with the bones, cartilage, and connective tissue of an animal like a chicken or larger animal like a cow or a pig. As that bone and cartilage are slow cooked at the right temperature over long periods, the collagen and other nutrients are boiled into the liquid. I know, I really hope no vegans just read that description. Putting that aside, and maybe trying not to think of exactly what is involved, look on this as the single best wonder drug available on the market today for better skin, stronger nails, healthier hair, and reduced cellulite. It contains multiple nutrients that are fantastic for your overall health, in particular, glucosamine, chondroitin, selenium, and iron. And you can make it in your kitchen!

Glucosamine is a natural compound found in the tissue that cushions the joints, which is the cartilage. It is often sold as supplements to reduce arthritis and inflammation. Together with Chondroitin, they have been shown to help improve joint health and is commonly taken by people suffering from osteoarthritis. Chondroitin is a vital part of the cartilage, and it is found naturally in the body. It gives the cartilage elasticity by retaining water because 65% to 80% of our cartilage is made up of water. As we age, that water retention decreases thus causing cartilage related problems like osteoarthritis.

Making your homemade bone broth is very easy - the hardest part may be sourcing the bones, but any reputable butcher will be able to give you these. Sometimes you might even find you will get them for free as they would only be throwing them out anyway, but with the rise in popularity of the keto diet, this might not last much longer! I always used to pretend that I had a dog I was getting the bones for, but I think the butcher started to get suspicious when I walked past his window multiple times per week and never walking a dog. The parts of the bone that are of particular importance are the cartilage, and the connective tissue as these are the parts that contain the collagen, so when selecting a bone, you ideally want one that has the highest concentration of these. Joints, knuckles, feet, and marrow bones are the juiciest and most suitable, and you can also use more meaty bones like short shank ribs to add flavor.

Primarily, the only elements needed to qualify for a bone broth are bones and water, but you can add meat and vegetables to that to create different tastes, textures, and results. Even though the usual delivery of bone broth is of a clear, slightly lumpy liquid, which is just derived straight from boiling the bones for long enough in hot water, there are plenty of ways that you can add in herbs or condiments to taste. In Chapter 6, I have included a 3-day bone broth fast for you to start to experience the benefits yourself, and I have done this in a way that you can make this your first three days of keto and combine your bone broth fast to combat the effects of keto flu.

I hope this chapter has given you a bit of an insight into exactly what bone broth is, what collagen is, and the fundamentals of the keto diet. In later chapters, we will be exploring these in more detail by looking at exactly why collagen is so important and delving much deeper into the best sources of collagen to add to your diet.

Chapter 2: Basics of Keto Diet

In the previous chapters, we looked at the general theory behind the keto diet, where it originated from, and we touched on the areas of collagen and bone broth. We will now look at the practical application of the keto diet into your lifestyle, what particular benefits it can bring to your overall health, and what results you can expect as part of your new lifestyle. Whenever you start any new diet or lifestyle transition, the information overload can be completely overwhelming, so I have tried to make this chapter in particular as easy to follow as possible by providing practical examples of how you can monitor and keep track of your ketosis levels. But the keto diet is by nature very technical, so if you find that this isn't something you are used to, start by using some of the tips in the 3-day plan to make sure that you have excellent preparation and organizing work done in advance.

As I mentioned in the last chapter, the keto diet is very firmly rooted in a scientific and holistic approach to your health. It requires a very delicate balance of food based on specific guidelines relating to the processing of fats and carbs in your system. Also, the way that you monitor ketones in your blood is part of a really focused process, which makes you take slightly more time to stop and consider your overall health. We will now look at that process in more detail.

The essential goal of the ketogenic diet is to increase the presence of ketones in your blood. In order to be sure that the diet is being effective and these ketones are present, there are two key ways that you can test for the presence of ketones in the comfort of your own home - breath analysis or urine analysis. I found the urine analysis ones a more cost-effective way to monitor my levels regularly, and once I got used to the process, it became effortless to do. You can buy urine test strips easily online through Amazon or at your local drug store, and there are now brands that are developed solely for use with the keto diet. They will come with a color chart on the side of the bottle to show you an easy reference guide on how to tell when you are in an active ketogenic metabolic state. As a rule, you want to be achieving 1.5-3 mmol/L of ketones present in your sample, and anything less than this would signify you are not currently operating in a keto state. By using these strips regularly, you can also monitor what types of foods instantly kick you out of your keto state, and you can adjust your intake accordingly.

Another useful product is a keto breath analyzer - again available through Amazon or maybe in your larger local drug stores and is around the same level of effectiveness as the keto urine strips. The other third way, which is probably considered the most effective, is by blood analysis - but for most people checking out the keto diet in order to lose weight, this is probably more invasive and unnecessary.

So now, you can work out how to tell when you are in the keto state, and we have also discussed more generally what the keto diet refers to. Now we will look much more specifically at what types of foods will put your body in the keto state, what the benefits are of being in this state, and how to incorporate a healthy keto diet into your daily routine.

The ketogenic diet is mainly based on the premise of a very delicate balance between carbs, fat, and protein. The commitment to ensuring the ratio of each is strictly monitored. For the Standard Ketogenic Diet (SKD), the recommended ratio is 75% fat, 20% protein and 5% carbs. That ratio is the basis for which the key metrics should be measured. With the Cyclical Ketogenic Diet (CKD), however, the ratio is determined over the week, with five keto days followed by two high carb days. And there is another option that allows you to increase your protein ratio, which is known as the High- Protein Ketogenic Diet, and the ratios are changed to 60% fat, 35% protein with still 5% carbs. Whichever one you decide to follow, I think you can at least agree that the terminology and measurement process involved in the keto lifestyle is certainly on another level from the usual "just eat fewer calories" dietary approach. So it is important for us to try and establish a few life hacks that help you keep on the right track with your keto goals.

When you first start your keto journey, you will most likely experience what is commonly known as the keto flu. Keto flu is your body's reaction to the sudden lack of the sugars and carbs that it has been used to running on. The symptoms will vary slightly for each person, but you will most likely start to feel extremely lethargic, with headaches, stomach issues such as constipation, and even nausea. Some people report feeling in a fog for a few days, and if you were particularly reliant on processed food and sugars, you might feel quite sluggish and not able to concentrate or think effectively for a few days. Try not to worry as these symptoms can sometimes present themselves very quickly. You should be able to combat this effectively with bone broth by following the advice in this book.

You may have noticed over the last few years the growth of the protein bar and protein supplement industry, and you will have plenty of packaged options screaming at you from the health aisle that they are completely safe to eat as part of your keto, paleo, or vegan diet. While some of these bars may, in fact, be ok for you to consume, please don't just trust the packaging and instead take some time to do research on the ingredients and also closely monitor your vitals before and after consuming so that you know the effect that it is having on your body. For example, some of the popular bars will be very high in sugar additives, and others will knock you out of the ketogenic state that you worked so hard to get in to. I'm sure you can imagine how frustrating it must be to eat a protein bar that clearly says keto-friendly and then realize that it has actually set you back on your journey, especially when you have spent the last three days drinking cartilage soup. So be careful, and when in doubt, don't buy it. I have included a recipe at the back of this book for almond butter bites that you can make yourself without any baking, and you will also be able to find numerous keto cookbooks online that can help in this area.

In this chapter, we took a bit more time to go over the keto diet and how to monitor your progress, and I hope that you are feeling confident and informed about your choice to use this dietary transition to transform your life. In the next chapter, we take another look at collagen and in particular, why it really matters and why it is so important to you at this stage of your keto journey.

Chapter 3: Is Collagen for you?

As we discussed earlier, when I first started my keto journey, I was disappointed at the level of information out there in particular reference to the use of bone broth in order to aid the symptoms of keto flu. I had discovered bone broth almost by accident and found it to be an almost 'miracle drug' through my first few days of carb detox. When I finally recovered from the flu-like symptoms, I took some time to research exactly why the bone broth had worked so well. I was surprised to discover the multi-faceted benefits of collagen that were contributing to making bone broth such a successful remedy. Thankfully I was pursuing this journey, much like yourself, at a time when collagen was a hot topic in the health and beauty industry. So, it really helped to have some influencers on YouTube and Instagram as well as regular health professionals in the media talking more about the benefits.

Collagen is the primary structural protein present in mammals, making it one of the most important types of protein found in our bodies. It is made up of amino acids that combine in such a way that they create a structure of strong connecting fibers throughout the body. Amino acids, and particularly the ones found in collagen, are imperative for the growth and strength of muscles, skin, hair, bone, and cartilage. As we grow older, the presence and strength of collagen decline - sometimes at a surprisingly rapid rate. Some amino acids are created naturally in the body until around the age of 25 and then starts to decline each year. You can expect to produce healthy levels of collagen until your early to mid-thirties, and by the time you enter your forties, your collagen levels will be noticeably reduced. When you think of all the areas of your body structure that collagen impacts, this timeline makes sense. Usually, as we age, our joints start to suffer, our skin loses its elasticity, and our hair and nails can become brittle and dull.

Every protein (including collagen) is made from building blocks known as amino acids. A sequence of these amino acids creates a polypeptide. A polypeptide can have a unique series of amino acids, which will help it perform a particular function. The sequence of amino acids in your DNA, for example, is different from that of collagen. It is fascinating to realize that even small changes in the series of amino acids can change the function and appearance of each protein so drastically.

So, what are amino acids? Amino acids are the building blocks of protein. Amino acids are organic compounds comprising of a sequence of carbon, hydrogen, oxygen, and nitrogen atoms. While all organic matter contains hydrogen, oxygen, and carbon, the addition of nitrogen sets protein apart. Scientists have identified over 500 amino acids in nature so far, but only 20 of them are present in human bodies. Of the thousands of different kinds of proteins found in the body, they are all built from various combinations of these 20 amino acids. These 20 amino acids are further classed into essential and non-essential amino acids. Essential amino acids are not produced in the human body, so they must be obtained from an external source like food. Non-essential amino acids can be produced by your body so eating foods that boost collagen will be beneficial. Explaining each amino acid will take another book, which is not the main point on why I wrote this book. Instead, I will talk about how you can get this into your diet and what benefits you can get from it.

Collagen is a popular commercial medical product used in cosmetic and restorative medical procedures. It can be used as natural tissue or be reconstructed artificially using animal tissue. Its versatility is key to its usefulness in medicine. Collagen can be reabsorbed. You can break it down, convert it to a different form, and the body can absorb it again. Collagen can exist in a solid form or a gel-like state. It can be used as a biomaterial or as part of a medical device. Collagen can come from cows, chickens, fish, pigs, or sheep.

Now that we have established how important it is, how do we improve and increase our collagen levels, and what exactly does it have to do with the ketogenic diet? One great way to get natural collagen into your body is through the consumption of bone broth. Bone broth is quite like a stock in the sense that it is the juices made from the cooking process of an animal, but bone broth is more specific in the way that it is cooked and hence the goodness and collagen content of it. By boiling animal bones in water for 24 hours or 12 hours for chicken bones, you are then left with a thick clear liquid when you remove the bone. The broth that is left after boiling will contain collagen as it has formed into gelatin that has been secreted from the bones throughout the process. This is a fantastic direct source of collagen and is also a tasty way to ensure you are getting nutrients without throwing yourself out of a ketogenic state.

The consumption of bone broth can also be of benefit to other aspects of your health. It can regulate your stomach acid, improve the protective lining within your gut, and it helps protect healthy gut bacteria, which are excellent for overall gut health. Combine that with the fact that it is also full of other essential nutrients that you need to be replenishing like potassium and calcium. Now you can start to see the benefits of this wonder drink. In older generations it was much more common to eat more of the animal as part of our diet and way back as hunters and gatherers there would have been literally nothing left after a hunt. So, if we look at the way our bodies are designed, then we can see how the modern diet and our modern lifestyle is working to actively starve us of some of the vital nutrients that we used to get naturally from our foods.

For pretty much every mineral or vitamin that you can think of, it is always better to consume in its natural state, but for various reasons, collagen is one that can be hard to find in its natural state in our modern diet. Particularly for vegetarians and vegans, the deficiency of this vital mineral can be an issue, and it is tough even to get the supplement form which is vegan-friendly due to the very nature of what collagen is. The purpose of this book is not to convince anyone of a particular lifestyle, it is only to confirm the benefits to those who are already doing or considering the keto lifestyle which is very much centered consuming meat.

I hope that helps to clarify some further details about the keto diet and the impact of collagen and the reasons behind why we might currently be struggling with a collagen deficiency. In the next chapter, we will look at the best sources of naturally occurring collagen.

Chapter 4: Best Sources of Collagen on a Keto Diet

In the last chapter, we looked in-depth at why collagen matters and why it makes up such a vital part of the recovery process when you start your journey with the keto diet. We also touched on why it can be so difficult to find naturally occurring in our modern foods and how to overcome this through the use of bone broth. In this chapter, I will be taking you through the process of sourcing as well as looking at other potential sources of collagen. One definite drawback of the best sources of collagen is that they don't accommodate a vegan lifestyle at all. Even collagen supplements are drawn from the bones of animals, so they will not be suitable for vegans. However, we will also look at other nutrients and vitamins that you can take to boost collagen production within your own body while still being able to adhere to a vegan or vegetarian lifestyle.

Although you can find great collagen supplements that will work to boost your collagen levels, it is certainly advisable, where possible, to get your collagen intake from food rather than supplements. This is because when your body digests the collagen in food or broth form, it can get straight to work and be absorbed more naturally into the body. If supplements are the only option available to you, though, they are certainly better than not getting the collagen, so please don't avoid taking them simply because they are not quite as effective as food-derived collagen.

Meat and fish are good sources of collagen and it is important how they are also consumed. For example, chicken is a fantastic source of collagen, but the best areas to consume are the chicken neck and cartilage, which may not be so regularly consumed. Again, that is what makes bone broth such an excellent choice as it allows you to get the full cartilage and collagen benefit but without having to eat it in its regular form. The same is true of fish, which again are a fantastic source of collagen but mostly if you eat the head and eyes. If you are reading this and feeling like that is all just a step too far for you then don't worry, it is possible to get these particular types of nutrients in supplement form, particularly eggshell membrane which can be dangerous to try and consume in its natural form if you value your veneers.

When you are sourcing meat, you have to be careful to buy only top quality and completely organic. This is because the nutrients that you are looking for in particular will only be present and of good quality in meat that has been well cared for, and hasn't been pumped full of water, additives or other chemicals. When you are buying beef, always look for grass-fed and organic because this will give the best quality meat. Also, look to purchase other cuts that might not be so readily popular and wherever possible try and buy from a local butcher or a farmer's market. When you purchase your meat directly from the farmers market or the butcher, not only can you be sure that the meat is fresh and of the best quality, but you also have an expert on hand to ask any questions to or discuss the particularly best cuts of meat that you want to be buying for your purpose. When buying chicken, always look for pasture-raised or free-range. It might seem like such a small adjustment, but even taking steps like these can be of huge benefit to the overall success of your new lifestyle.

There are some foods that, although might not be direct sources of collagen, can contribute to overall collagen levels because they contain key ingredients such as Vitamin C and Proline, which plays an important role in collagen synthesis. You can get Vitamin C from lemons, bell peppers, kale, and red cabbage. These will work actively to help your body produce collagen, thereby naturally increasing collagen levels. All of these foods are also keto-friendly, so you can enjoy packing as much of them into your diet as you can, safe in the knowledge that you are boosting your exposure to collagen at the same time. In the recipes in Chapter 6, I have included examples of how to include foods like this into your diet. You can also use mushrooms as a great alternative to meat - for example using the cap of a large portobello mushroom for a veggie burger actually gives the same texture as meat would and can be seasoned very similar. Obviously, if you are having a burger, make sure you are not having a bun and instead try wrapping it in two iceberg lettuce leaves in order to keep it keto.

Tropical fruits and berries are excellent to boost collagen, but you have to be very careful with the keto diet that you don't consume too much fruit as it is high in carbs and can kick you out of the keto state. My advice would be to stick to blueberries and lemons in moderation, or you can treat yourself to avocado with eggs for your breakfast meal since avocados are high in fat and a bit of a keto superfood, but other than that you should be looking at more vegetable and meat-based alternatives for suitable sources of collagen. Lemon infused water is a great health drink and you can keep it in the refrigerator chilling overnight, to be taken out in the morning and provide you with a drink packed with the vitamins of the lemons without worrying about having to consume the fruit.

If you are following a vegan or vegetarian diet and want to try keto, it is tough, but it is possible. Actually, it is very similar in the way it follows the fat, protein, and carb ratios, but this time, all of the fat and protein have to be found from non-animal sources. We have already spoken about how some vegetables and fruits are naturally occurring slow carbs, and you can also get plant-based fats and plant-based proteins. But with this diet, you will have to pretty much solely rely on supplements in order to get the vital minerals like B12, iron, zinc, and collagen. Remove any grains from your diet. Your food will instead need to be packed with leafy greens, high protein vegan "meat" such as non-GMO tofu, mushrooms, and vegetables like zucchini, cauliflower, and broccoli. And substitute any dairy as usual with items like coconut or almond milk. This book is not intended as a guide for the vegan or vegetarian keto diet, and if this is the route you decide to take I would suggest trying to find some additional resources to help you really analyze the types of foods and nutrients that you need to be consuming.

I hope I have given you useful information on how to source collagen, get clean keto ingredients, and what foods you can consume. You will learn about making your own bone broth at home in the next chapter.

Chapter 5: How to Make Bone Broth

We have talked about the importance of bone broth and why it is such a miracle "cure-all" for the transition to the keto lifestyle and for the keto flu in particular. In this chapter, I want to go into detail about how to actually make bone broth, what you will need to prepare in advance, and the suggested quantities to use for this. If you want to cheat, you can purchase pre-made and pre-packaged bone broth either online or at reputable health food stores. However, if you have extra time, I would strongly recommend you make your own. I have included details below, which will hopefully make this a lot easier for you. Part of the keto lifestyle is going to involve some additional lifestyle changes, so the more food that you can prepare and cook from scratch, the more significant the difference you will see to your overall health and wellbeing.

Bone broth is such a traditional recipe that it may take a while for you to get used to actually having to buy bones to cook with. In previous generations, when this was much more popular, the bone broth was made with leftover carcasses from the meat. Modern meat preparation methods usually absolve us from having to deal with this part of the process, but now that you know you will require bones for your bone broth, one simple adjustment you can start making is to buy meat on the bone more often. Buy whole chickens instead of just chicken breast and purchase more unusual joints of meat such as knuckles, joints and feet, and bone marrow. Your shopping cart will start to look a little different, but this is all part of the new life adjustment. Once you begin to incorporate making the broth into your weekly routine, you will soon get used to the changes.

For the flavoring of the bone broth, you can select as many herbs and add as many green vegetables as you like, but some work particularly well. The bone broth will always have a very strong meaty, almost greasy flavor, so try and bring in some fresh herbs like thyme or parsley. Ashwagandha is another one that works particularly well and is a bit of a superfood in itself as it is known to boost brain function - that will come in very useful during the fog of the keto flu! When you are selecting which vegetables to use, another great way is to keep your vegetable scraps like broccoli stalk, butt ends of onions, carrots, or celery. You can put them in a container, freeze, and then defrost them when you decided to make a bone broth. You can, of course, use fresh vegetables if you like.

Now, while the idea of rustic scrap bones and leftover vegetables is quite reassuringly authentic, we also have to make sure that you are still taking care of your health and not accidentally consuming anything that is bad for you. For this reason, it is strongly advisable only to purchase organic or grass-fed beef and take some time before preparing the bone broth to roast it first.

The recipe below will give you around 16 cups of bone broth and takes around 10 minutes to prepare. Bone broth by nature takes time to cook because the bones need time to really marinate and excrete all the goodness into the broth, so you would want to prepare this at least the in the morning and allowing about 12 to 24 hours of total cooking time. The recommended consumption for bone broth is 3-4 cups per day, but for your first few days of the keto flu, you can be drinking a few more than this to keep you going.

You will need:

 2 pounds of grass-fed beef bones or free-range chicken bones
 1-gallon water - cold
 1 onion

2 carrots

2 stalks of celery

3 tbsp apple cider vinegar

2 cloves of garlic

Herbs and spices to taste

Salt and pepper to taste

A small bunch of parsley as garnish

1. Preheat the oven to 350F° and prepare all your bones in a roasting pan.

2. Roast the bones in the oven for around 35 minutes.

3. Remove the bones from the oven and transfer to a large stockpot.

4. Add the cold water and the apple cider vinegar to the pot and leave to sit for 30 minutes.

5. While the bones are cooling in the water, you can use the time to prepare your vegetables. Whether you are using scraps or fresh vegetables, chop them to roughly similar sizes.

6. Add your vegetables, herbs and spices, salt and pepper into the large pot, and bring the whole mixture to the boil, stirring regularly.

7. Once the broth has started to boil, reduce the heat and simmer for at least 12 hours.

8. Check the mixture regularly, maybe around every hour, and you might find that a foamy. layer starts to appear - you can remove this from the broth with a spoon.

9. When the broth is nearly ready, add in the garlic and the parsley, and simmer for around another 30 minutes.

10. Once the broth is ready, remove from the heat and allow the whole mixture to cool.

11. Pour over a fine strainer into large freezer-proof storage jars. If you spread the mixture over. five jars, that will give you one for every weekday, and you can freeze or refrigerate as necessary.

This will give you a large quantity of bone broth on standby, which is great to have for ensuring you are fully prepared for the week. When you are ready to consume the bone broth, pour the mixture from one of the jars into a saucepan, boil, and then transfer into a mug. Enjoy!

Chapter 6: 3-Day Keto Collagen Diet Plan

When I was first learning about the benefits of the ketogenic diet and the particular benefits of bone broth and collagen, I tried hard to find specific meal plans to help with the transition. There are lots of helpful resources online when it came to keto in general, but I wanted to really focus on the implementation of collagen in my diet, and I found that there was not so much information online concerning this. For that reason, I decided to develop my own 3-day collagen and bone broth diet plan. This incorporates all three mealtimes. I have also included details in other chapters about Intermittent Fasting. If you are doing time-restricted feeding, you can reduce this to two meals instead. I have tried everything from the extremes of drinking nothing but bone broth for days to eating only eggs for every meal - trust me when I say you definitely want to be having some variety in both those diets!

I want to save you from having to go through the same ordeal I did in finding the right combination of food and fasting that worked for me. I prepared this 3-day Keto Collagen recipe and meal plan guide to help. The great thing about adding more collagen to your keto diet is that it will actually open you up to more foods. If you have already made the decision to go keto and you are now trying to find a way to increase the levels of collagen, then this plan will work by hopefully giving you some great alternatives to add to your diet. And if you are brand new to the ketogenic diet and are just about to start, the 3-day plan below will help you get through the keto flu better than a lot of other programs out there. In the final chapter, I talk a bit about the journaling process and how this helped me in particular throughout this three-day stretch. Please check it out, and I would strongly recommend that as part of your preparation. You will find some key metrics to monitor so that you can ensure your physical, mental, and emotional health throughout this process. It is unlikely that you will have any adverse reactions, as long as you are in good physical shape when you start. But as with any dietary life change, it would be worth consulting with your doctor first.

Bone Broth Fast

Bone broth works at its best when it is incorporated with Intermittent Fasting, commonly known as the bone broth fast. So don't worry if you thought you were going to have to consume nothing but bone broth for three days, it's not quite that bad. I have covered much more on the area of intermittent fasting in the last chapter, but for now, let me give you a quick introduction to what we mean by intermittent fasting and also describe how it will prove crucial to your first few days of keto. We will then start to look at examples of how we combine these two areas of bone broth and fasting in order to supercharge our results. Fasting has long been recognized as a great way to not only regulate and rid your body of toxins but also to help with illnesses. We start to understand this a bit better when we consider just how much energy is taken up in our bodies by the digestive system. It is almost half. That means half of the energy we consume is then used to digest that consumption of the energy. Then when we add in the fact that most people will have breakfast within an hour of waking and probably eat an evening meal around an hour or two before bed, your digestive system is literally working from morning until night.

Combine that with all the energy that your body naturally needs to allow you to work out, run errands, go to the office, concentrate, and have memory function, all of these other tasks that we take for granted but which are regularly expending energy. That doesn't leave a lot of energy for dealing with whole-body maintenance, cell regeneration, or healing of damaged cells. By extending the time that we don't eat by even just a few hours per day, we allow our body to use some of the energy that it would have been spending on digestion to go to work repairing and healing our bodies. This is why fasting states are so important.

There are two ways to approach fasting - some people fast for one day a week or one weekend a month, and while this is great for the system, it can be quite hard to maintain. An easy way to incorporate the benefits of fasting is by bringing it into your everyday routine, and simply extending the time period within which you don't eat and shortening the time period within which you do eat. This is why the bone broth fast works so well because even during the fasting periods, you can consume collagen filled bone broth, which will regulate your energy levels but not kick you out of your keto state. Simple!

After a few days, you become so adjusted to the state that you no longer feel hungry outside your eating window and you can start to notice benefits like clearer skin, improved concentration, and memory and even reduced anxiety or depression symptoms. It really can be a miracle way to control your diet. The easiest way to do this would be to skip breakfast and only eat between late morning and early evening - anything from 4 to 8 hours of eating is optimum. Incorporating bone broth into your fasting times works not only to relieve the symptoms of hunger but also to increase the all-important levels of collagen that are getting into your system.

You can have bone broth as much as you like during your fasted time window as it is not going to end your fast, but it is also much more beneficial than just drinking regular water as it is flooding your body with much-needed collagen. For these reasons, I have incorporated the bone broth fast into your handy three-day meal plan to kickstart your keto journey by suggesting times for you to consume the broth.

Preparation

It is important, first of all, to think about what we are going to need in advance. With any change of lifestyle and change of diet, there is usually the need for a kitchen overhaul. I would strongly advise getting rid of any foods that you currently have which are not suitable for keto. Over the next three days, you are going to crave carbs and sugar so much that it would just be too tempting for you if you had that type of food lying around. As we mentioned in a previous chapter, if you really cannot get over your initial cravings for sugar, then try small pieces of keto-friendly protein bars, snack on fruit, or have a cup of bone broth. The most important thing is not to end up accidentally consuming so much sugar or carbs that you kick yourself out of the keto state. These three days will be intense if you have been living a life mostly consisting of processed food, alcohol, and takeaways. It might be a good idea to try it over a weekend when you have less work to do, or work from home and spend the time really being able to focus on what you are putting into your body.

Once you have completely cleared your cupboards and emptied your fridge (especially of alcohol!), then it is time to start prepping for the shopping list for your new life. You might also want to consider purchasing some new kitchen equipment - you don't have to, but if you decide that this is going to be a lifestyle change for you, then there will be certain items that will be particularly handy to have around the kitchen. Items such as a blender, spiralizer, slow cooker, BPA-free storage containers, and drinking cups would all help with the adjustments to your new eating routine. These are not necessary because mostly everything contained below can be made without the use of these items, so don't worry if you do not possess these yet.

Day One

Breakfast

When you first wake up, try and start your day with some water to flush out your system and wait at least three hours after waking to have any form of food. Over the next three days, we will be extending this even further, so enjoy your breakfast, especially today! For day one, it would be a great idea to have an egg-based dish for your breakfast to keep you extra full for the day ahead. Remember and be extra mindful of how you are cooking your eggs, remember that you need to make sure you are using olive oil, and if making scrambled eggs you are switching to keto-friendly, unsweetened coconut or almond milk. If you are feeling really adventurous and still full of energy on day one, then try my tasty breakfast burrito recipe below, which is enough for one serving of a healthy breakfast burrito.

You will need:

    2 large eggs, organic

    1 tbsp coconut cream

    1 tsp chili flakes

    1 tsp fresh rosemary

    1 tbsp olive oil

1. Whisk the eggs together in a bowl along with the coconut cream, and add in the chili flakes and rosemary as you go.
2. Heat the oil in a pan, and once ready add in the mixture above.
3. The goal is to make a stable omelet shape which will serve as the wrap for your burrito so. make sure that you cook thoroughly and flip halfway through cooking.
4. Serve with your choice of toppings and salt and pepper to taste.

Once you have this base, you can add any toppings that you want, then fold into a burrito shape. My personal favorites are avocado, bacon, and a touch of spinach, but the great thing with this recipe is that you can throw in as many keto-friendly additions as you like. The more you change it up, the more you can have it as a regular breakfast staple that the whole family will enjoy. And the eggs and avocados are particularly great sources of collagen to kick start your day.

Lunch

Before lunch, you can have some bone broth as a late morning or early afternoon snack so that by lunchtime, you are not completely starving, and can just have something light. The ideal is to have prepared something the night before that you can quickly heat up in the office microwave, or even better if you have leftovers of some protein and collagen-rich foods that you made for last night's meal.

If you have the time to cook something from scratch though check out my keto chicken noodle recipe below which will be enough for around two regular servings

You will need:

>   1 lb cabbage - thinly sliced into strips
>
>   ¼ cup onions - thinly sliced
>
>   2 cloves garlic - thinly sliced
>
>   2 tbsp olive oil

1. Heat the oil in a pan, and then add in the mixture of ingredients.
2. Sauté the cabbage, onions, and garlic until the garlic becomes translucent and the cabbage is tender - this should probably take around ten minutes.

Once this is ready, you have a fantastic cabbage noodle base available for you to add any grilled protein topping that you want. Grilled chicken or pan-fried salmon go particularly well, and then you have a healthy, keto-friendly, collagen packed lunch in less than twenty minutes.

Snack

Throughout the afternoon, try and avoid snacking as much as possible. If you need to, make sure that anything you are eating is keto-friendly, and always try and consume as much bone broth as you can to try and control your cravings. On day one, you probably want to aim for around 3-4 cups of bone broth throughout your day, and you will really notice the benefits to your energy levels. If you feel like you know in advance that you might need some sugary treats to get you through the day, then try my recipe below for homemade almond butter bars. You can carry this with you throughout the day and know that you can enjoy a healthy snack that will still allow you to stay within the limits of your keto diet.

You will need:

2 cups Collagen infused almond butter

½ cup keto-friendly maple syrup (monk fruit maple syrup is 100% keto friendly)

¾ cup coconut flour

¼ cup of water - you might not need this but be ready just in case

1. Combine the collagen-infused almond butter, the keto-friendly maple syrup, and the coconut flour in a mixing bowl.

2. Mix until the mixture becomes pliable, and if you find at times that it is getting too tough, you can add drops of the water to soften it slightly.

3. Once you have the mixture smooth and shapeable, you can start to make the small bar shapes that you want.

4. Wrap each individual bar in parchment paper and put them in the refrigerator to set. This should take around 30-45 minutes.

Once they have set, you can now safely enjoy a delicious treat throughout your day, and no baking was even involved! The above recipe should give you 4-6 bars depending on how large you make them, feel free to adjust the recipe so that you can make more.

Dinner

On day one, try and think about bringing the timing of your evening meal slightly earlier, certainly at least four hours before going to sleep. In this way, you increase the period of your fasting window. After your evening meal, you can keep your energy levels up and your hunger satiated with some bone broth or herbal tea.

After your first full day of following the keto diet, you will be craving a great meal, so I have included two meals below.

Mexican stuffed peppers with grass-fed beef

You will need:

4 large bell peppers

1 pound of ground organic, grass-fed beef

½ onion - thinly chopped

1 clove garlic - thinly sliced

1 tsp cumin, 1 tsp chili powder

½ cup tomato puree

2 tbsp olive oil

1. Cut four large peppers in half from their stalk to their stem, lie on their back and remove the core and seeds.
2. Place them on their backs in a baking tray.
3. Meanwhile, preheat the oven at 350F°.
4. Heat the oil in a pan, then add the onions and garlic, sauté until onions start to brown and the garlic starts to become translucent.
5. Add in the ground beef, cook until the beef begins to brown, then add the seasoning along with salt and pepper to taste.
6. Once the beef is ready, spoon the mixture into the open pepper shells and then bake the entire meal in the oven for around twenty-five minutes.

Wild-caught salmon or organic chicken with zucchini noodles

Salmon is a fantastic collagen-boosting food that should be enjoyed on a keto diet. However, you will also need to be careful about the origins of the food that you are eating, as we discussed previously in the book. For that reason, wild-caught salmon is always optimal, and be sure to do your research about where to buy the freshest fish and meat produce in your local area.

For the zucchini noodles, it would be easier to make, especially if you took my advice and invested in that spiralizer. And because they are made of zucchini, you can cook them similar to normal noodles, and they can be enjoyed either hot or cold.

You will need:

4 salmon fillets

2 zucchinis, spiralized

Extra virgin olive oil

2 tsp. minced garlic

1 lemon

¼ onion

Sea salt or himalayan salt

Black pepper

1 bunch of parsley (optional)

1. Season salmon with salt and pepper and set aside.
2. Spiralize the zucchinis using a spiralizer to make the noodles.
3. Drain the zucchini noodles and pat dry with paper towels and set aside.
4. In a pan, heat 1 tbsp of olive oil and sear the salmon on each side. Transfer to a plate and let it rest.
5. In the same pan, heat 1 tbsp of olive oil and add the lemon slices to deglaze the pan.
6. Stir fry the onion, garlic, and noodles for about 5 minutes until the noodles are al dente.
7. Serve the noodles with salmon on top.
8. Season with salt and pepper.

9. Garnish with parsley (optional).

Make sure you follow the instructions for preparing your salmon and then add the noodles to your plate to make it a full meal. Remember that leafy greens can be consumed in any quantity with your meals, so be sure to make a nice salad that can be added to any plate, and instead of using a dressing, try adding a small amount of apple cider vinegar.

Dessert

And since you have probably been struggling with day one of the transitions to your new diet, I will even be extra generous and allow you to have a dessert on day one. Just remember the important thing about these three days is to reduce the amount of time that you actually spend eating, so just make sure that dessert is finished at least four hours before you go to bed. Since tomorrow morning might feel quite long as we extend the fasting window, I would advise having your dinner a lot earlier than usual and then giving yourself a bit of a break before dessert. Learning to space out meals and manage hunger is a large part of the keto diet also.

Baking your own keto-friendly desserts can require a complete kitchen overhaul in terms of flour and sugars, so while you are still getting used to the diet, try and stick to some easier alternatives. The almond bars that you made above are a perfect way to end the meal or prepare a superfood bowl with some avocados, raspberries, and blackberries.

In the guidelines for day two and three, I will focus less on recipes and more on the types of food you will be eating, but I hope that handy guide for day one really set you up well.

Day Two

For day two, we want to be pushing your fasting window even longer, so you want to try and have a cup of bone broth in the morning and then wait around 5 hours from waking before you have your breakfast. For breakfast, I would suggest a vegetable-packed green juice - being sure to add a touch of collagen powder to it also, and adding in greens like spinach, cucumber, celery, and kale. Usually, when making this type of green juice you would be using a cored apple as the juice base, but apples are a no go for keto due to the percentage of sugar they contain, so swapping that out for just plain water will allow the greens to mix well and protect your blades slightly. When you first start with this diet, you might struggle to believe that it is possible to start your whole day without a proper breakfast, but packing this much veggie content into your first meal will set your day up for success in the right way.

For the bone broth fast, it is important to have a short eating window and a long fasting window, so for example if you naturally wake up at 7 am, then don't eat until 12noon, then be sure to finish your evening meal by 6 pm, and that gives you an 18 hour fasting and 6 hour eating window which is absolutely optimal for the benefits you are looking for.

If you can get to this stage on day two, that's fantastic, but if you need one more day to adjust then, that's fine to leave it until day three. Just make sure you have plenty of bone broth ready so that you are minimizing the feeling of fasting because you are able to have some cups of broth to keep you going.

Since you had such a large dinner last night and will no doubt have some meat and fresh greens leftover, I would suggest packing yourself a nice healthy and substantial lunch full of everything that was left. Also, you can cook up small amounts of cauliflower rice to add to your lunch in order to make it a bit more filling or to make it seem like a whole different meal instead of just leftovers from the previous night. You can always consider adding in extra keto superfoods like broccoli or asparagus, as a substitute to any high carb foods you would usually have there.

Throughout the day on day two, you can have your almond butter bites that you made. Remember also that it is important to adjust to the keto diet as a new way of eating and consuming food. Although you can have these treats in order to help you adjust, you do want to be transitioning to the stage where your taste buds now appreciate the no sugar parts of your diet, and you are used to much larger meat and veg portions for each meal. Evening meal on day two should still be packed full of protein and leafy greens, and for an extra boost of collagen, be sure to add garlic, bell peppers, or walnuts into as many recipes as you can.

Remember to have some bone broth in the evening in order to get that extra boost of collagen for the day. Always drink lots of water as you are going through this process. It will not only help keep you hydrated and keep you from getting severe withdrawal headaches but will also help deter hunger pangs and allow you to transition better to your fasting regime.

Day Three

By this point, you might be feeling the real effects of the keto flu - so be sure to have plenty of bone broth ready for the mornings, to help you stay in a fasting state for longer. For day three, we are not going to have any breakfast at all, and from today onwards, you want to really be keeping your eating window to 6 hours and consuming your meals between those times.

Same as yesterday, try and make your first meal of the day packed with leafy greens, so consuming them in a juice is a great way to achieve this while still being able to fit it around a busy lifestyle. Some people on the keto diet also start having steak and eggs for breakfast, and if you can incorporate this in your schedule and it suits you to do so, please feel free. We are looking at changes and additions to your day that can be incorporated over long periods, so really try and make sure that you are consuming as wide a variety of foods as possible. And maybe save the steak for your evening meal.

Try to bring in more plant-based meals by day three, perhaps a portobello mushroom burger, or you can make noodles from zucchini, or try and improve the variety of salad bowls that you are eating by mixing it up with some sunflower seeds, sliced almonds or pepitas. The key is to try foods that are outside your comfort zone and get used to new textures and new tastes, and then find the ones that you like then keep those as you transition this three-day bootcamp style plan into a long-lasting lifestyle change.

In the evening of day three, remember to keep pushing through when it comes to the symptoms of the flu - keep drinking your infused water, taking your supplements, and drinking those all-important cups of bone broth.

You have done so well to get to this stage, and because of that, I want to congratulate you. Congratulations on successfully completing three days of your brand new diet! Considering the large quantity of processed food and sugar that was in my diet when I went through the keto flu, I'm surprised I actually survived the three days! So no matter how tough the transition was for you, I completely understand, and I'm very proud of you for making it this far. In the next chapter, I have included some wider lifestyle tips that will help you cement this as part of your journey and add in some great habits to help you along the way. It has been such a privilege being your guide. I'm happy to be able to now lead you into some more enjoyable parts of your new healthy lifestyle.

Chapter 7: Next Steps

Congratulations on completing your 3-day ketogenic diet plan! You will now hopefully be completely rid of the symptoms of keto flu, and should already be starting to see some of the new benefits to this new lifestyle. Depending on just how much of a change this new diet was compared to your old food choices, you have either spent the last 3 days with a slightly sore head and being a bit more snappy than usual, or you have been unable to get out of bed, walk more than five steps or even raise your arm without feeling exhausted. The more you needed to detox, the worse it would have been. The great thing is though that now the worst is over. Welcome to your new life!

You will, by now, have a great appreciation for just how much your body was ruled by the things that you were eating. Hopefully, the study of this subject has also taught you a lot more about your body and how you are impacted by every food choice that you make. There is so much more to living a healthy lifestyle than just cutting out carbs, so in this chapter I just wanted to take some time to touch on a few other areas of wellness that you should now be looking to incorporate into your daily life, to ensure your success on this journey. We will look into the areas of incorporating a solid morning routine, exercise, herbs, supplements, and intermittent fasting - all of which, when used appropriately, can add substantial gains to your keto goals.

Supplements

Incorporating supplements into your daily diet is going to be vitally important throughout your transition process with keto, and probably beyond that as well. MCT Oil is a great choice to start and can be purchased very easily in most health food stores. MCT is metabolized in your system slightly differently than other nutrients, so it allows for better absorption into your blood, therefore resulting in being an efficient and clean energy source for your muscles and brain functions. Add a teaspoon of oil to any shakes, smoothies or salad for a quick energy boost. MCT is also found naturally in coconut oil, so be sure to add this in regular quantities to your diet, as well as using coconut oil for cooking.

Magnesium is another excellent supplement with multiple benefits when engaging with a keto-friendly diet. Taken in pill form, and available widely at health food stores, magnesium is an excellent supplement for the promotion of healthy bones and joints and will help relieve muscle cramps, which you may be experiencing as part of your keto flu. It also regulates your blood sugar levels and thereby helping to regulate your energy levels, so it would be advisable to make this a regularly added supplement to your diet. There are some keto-friendly, magnesium-rich foods like spinach and avocado, but taking a supplement does not mean that you should remove these foods from your diet.

As you adapt to your diet being completely different and to having to eliminate most of the sugary tastes from your diet, you can find that a great way to ease this transition is to stock up on keto-friendly protein bars. There are some great brands out there, and as long as they are consumed in the right quantities. Always check the ingredients and make sure that you are buying snacks that use real ingredients. The important thing is that you educate yourself on being able to tell whether they are suitable for you based on reading and understanding the packaging. When in doubt, leave it out. Some of the popular brands on the market will contain unhealthy sugar substitutes that you don't want to be consuming. This is also why it is important to regularly test your ketosis levels, as it can depend on your body weight and some other factors whether something might tip you just over the edge and out of ketosis. So even though these types of bars claim to be keto-friendly, do your research on how they impact your own body before making them a staple part of your diet.

It is important to remember that most protein bars will also have a high carb content, so don't buy something just because it says it is high in protein. You also want to be checking that the bar is keto-friendly and has a low level of carbs. Most supplements, energy bars or shakes in the wellness industry will have a note on the packaging whether they are paleo-friendly, keto-friendly, or vegan-friendly. Such is the awareness now of these distinct dietary areas that you will start noticing this type of packaging more often.

Exercise

If you thought you had managed to get through the whole book without a good old-fashioned lecture on the benefits of exercise, then I'm so sorry to disappoint! In all seriousness though, we all know the importance of exercise and when you are embarking on a significant lifestyle change such as the ketogenic diet, you would be doing yourself a disservice if you didn't also try and work hard to at least bring in a small element of a daily exercise routine into your life. Exercise doesn't have to be disruptive to your day. In the next section, we will cover how to make sure that keto is appropriately managed with a structured routine, so this is a fantastic opportunity to include in that some structure around when and how you work out.

Small changes can make the biggest difference. I want to stay away from recommending "keto-friendly" exercises as really there are no wrong exercises to do at any time. While you are adjusting to your new diet, try and avoid most high-intensity workouts and extreme classes like cross-fit or spin. You can build up to these, but while your body is in the transition process it is advisable to stick to regular cardio such as walking or jogging, and even better to do some yoga.

Strength workouts are fantastic for toning your body and building muscle instead of fat, and you should aim to have a good 20-30 minutes of this type of workout at least twice a week. When doing strength workouts with keto, try and stick to low weights and do more repetitions. Be sure to stay extra hydrated as well as keeping a regular note of how you feel after your workouts, in case you need to start adding in extra supplements or protein powder.

Daily Routine

Being disciplined about a good daily routine is essential to the long-term success of any dietary change. The more structured and organized your day is, the more likely you are to stay on track with any significant diet adjustments. Particularly for the first few days and weeks of keto, you might find the cravings at times overwhelming, so by packing your morning with some key non-negotiables is an effective way to ensure you are more likely to follow through on your plan. You will also be doing a lot of extra preparatory work for the foods that you will be eating, and you will likely be using cooking methods that you have not experienced before. It is important, therefore, to give yourself adequate time throughout your day but particularly in the morning to master all of the new skills that you will need.

Before we look in-depth at a great morning routine, it is also important to ensure you are getting quality sleep. Ideal sleep times are between 9 pm and 6 am, so while it might sound impossible right now, the ideal way to wake up in the morning is without an alarm clock and actually either before or with the natural rising of the sun. The benefits of this can be extraordinary and it also says more about your mindset and your consistency when you get into a strict sleep and waking routine. Consistency and a strong mindset will be very useful tools as you commence a keto lifestyle.

When we sleep, as well as processing all the important information of the day, our brain works on filing short- and long-term memories. It decides which memories and learned experiences from throughout the waking day are useful to keep and which ones we can forget. It is strongly advisable not to use your phone for at least an hour before bed and to remove all screens from the bedroom. The blue light that is emitted from screens is disruptive to our brains and to the parts of our processing centers that are required to wind down before sleeping because it is on a constant state of alertness due to whatever we are watching at the time.

Once you have mastered the art of getting up without an alarm clock, there are a couple of habits that you should be looking to do for the first hour that you are awake, and absolutely none of them will require looking at your phone. The last hour before we sleep and the first hour we wake are the two most important areas of the day. So it is vitally important that you build in a strong exercise, meditation, and mindfulness routine for the first hour of waking, to prepare yourself properly mentally and physically for the day ahead. This is also an excellent time to prep for your meals, and as you adjust to the new eating plans, you will be grateful for the additional time in the morning to plan out what to eat for the day.

Journal Your Progress

A good habit that I got into while preparing for the transition to keto was to monitor my physical, mental, and emotional states as much as possible by keeping a detailed health journal. Establishing baseline measurements for most of the data that I would be recording like urine ketone levels and resting heart rate was valuable. It also helped get me in the practice of really taking time out every day to analyze how I was feeling and to record any changes. Even if, at the time, I wasn't sure what was causing them. I was able to look back in this journal, identify obvious food, sleep, or exercise triggers that were actually causing changes in my mood and my behavior.

Once I had been able to establish a pattern, I was then able to use that data to help me get through the significant changes that were happening in the first few days of keto flu. Logging which symptoms I felt at which time enabled me to check back and see what helped and what didn't, and it is from that analysis that I prepared the 3-day keto collagen meal plan. I would advise that you take the time to monitor the changes in your body and be aware of what factors will affect your mood. Prepare in advance for the times when you know you are going to lose concentration, perhaps, feel a bit down or not be motivated and make sure that you have some remedies handy in order to overcome it.

Intermittent Fasting (IF)

The easiest way to implement IF is to remove early breakfast and late-night snacks from your menu completely. Looking first of all at an IF schedule of 16 hours fasting and 8 hours eating - you would wake up at 6 am and only drink water until around 10 or 11 am. You would then have a late breakfast or have your lunch around 1 or 2 pm, and then you can have your evening meal around 5 or 6 pm as long as you are finished eating for 6 or 7 pm. There are several schools of thought when it comes to what drinks you can have outside of these times and a lot of people (myself included) would not be able to make it until 11 am without some form of caffeine. If you feel like you really need something in the morning, then stick to black coffee or green tea. And at night before you go to bed, stick to non-caffeinated drinks such as chamomile tea. You can drink water at all times and actually the more water you drink, the better.

The thinking behind IF is that your digestive system actually uses up so much energy digesting your food that it never really gets the chance during waking hours to redirect any of that energy to other parts of the body that may require healing. By effectively starving your system in very short doses, it allows your digestive system to quiet down and for your body to heal and renew itself much more effectively. The results of IF are staggering, and I would strongly suggest this is something that you try yourself.

If you are feeling extremely adventurous, start with 8/16 (8 hours of eating window) and work your way down to 4/20. The schedule for this could be to wake up at 6 am, have some black coffee, drink water throughout the morning and then have lunch at 12 noon, a small snack around 2 pm and an early dinner just before 4 pm. These times can be pushed back if you prefer an evening meal. Now, if you have never heard of this before, I bet you are looking at those times and saying that it is impossible for you ever to be able to implement something so extreme into your life. The hunger that you feel most of the time is a conditioned response in your brain. You have a brilliant and resilient body, and it will very quickly learn these new eating windows. You will soon find you no longer wake up hungry, and actually, you are consuming much less over a daily period. This also helps massively with the dreaded afternoon slump.

As with all new diets, please consult your doctor before trying the extreme version of this, especially if you are currently taking any medication. Incorporating an 8/16 version should be a very healthy alternative for you. And one of the huge benefits of following this type of time-restricted eating is that you generally get more leeway with what foods you are allowed to eat during your eating periods. That is definitely not the case with the keto diet. Unfortunately, you will need to make sure you are still sticking to the strict boundaries of the ketogenic rules, so it might be a good idea to extend your eating window just to be sure.

Once your system gets used to the new routine, which should only take a few days, you will notice that the hunger pangs have gone, particularly in the morning. Throughout your shortened eating window, you also get fuller much faster, and as a result, don't end up eating so much that you are left with a bloated feeling. All in all, it works in alignment with the basic requirements of your system and you should start to feel the impact of having all that extra energy left to flush out the toxins and regenerate the cells in the rest of your body.

Final Words

Wow - you made it! I was sure that I might have lost you when I first started talking about the cartilage soup, so I'm absolutely delighted that you made it all the way to the finish line! I hope you have enjoyed this journey into the world of collagen and keto diet. I hope that you have survived your first few days of keto flu and are now fully over your symptoms and feeling much better about this fantastic new lifestyle choice. When I first started my keto journey, there wasn't as much readily available information as there now is, so I hope that I have added a particular style of voice to the keto community. I really appreciate the opportunity to have been able to share my story.

Throughout this book, we have looked at the good, the bad, and the often ugly, but underneath all of the great advice and the strategies lies the commitment that you have made to take that first step into the unchartered water towards transforming your life. That is what the ketogenic diet can do - it can transform your body, your health, and your mind by cutting out toxins such as sugar, alcohol, and reducing carbs and grains Your internal system will be running like a well-tuned sports car. You will be starting to feel the benefits of greater clarity, improved cognitive functioning, deeper sleep, more energy, and that all-important drop in the numbers on the scale.

I wish you the best of luck with the continuation of your journey because there is always so much more to learn and it doesn't end here. There is a fantastic community out there of which this is just one small part, and I would encourage you to engage with as many of the health practitioners, influencers and community builders that you can find. In doing so, I hope you find your tribe that will support you for the rest of this journey.

Thanks again for allowing me to be a small part of your story so far, and best of luck with the rest of your ketogenic lifestyle

www.ingramcontent.com/pod-product-compliance
Lightning Source LLC
Chambersburg PA
CBHW031301250726
48655CB00005B/2300